# How to lose weight:
## A complete solution to weight loss and weight  maintenance problems

# Table of contents


Chapter1

Chapter2

Chapter3

Chapter4

Chapter1

# Simple ways that aid in weight loss

## 1. Do not miss breakfast

Skipping breakfast will not help you lose weight. You might miss out on crucial nutrients and you may wind up nibbling more during the day because you feel hungry.

## 2. Eat frequent meals

Eating at regular periods throughout the day helps burn calories at a quicker pace. It also lessens the impulse to munch on meals heavy in fat and sugar.

Find out more about eating healthily

## 3. Eat lots of fruit and veg

Fruit and veg are low in calories and fat, and rich in fiber - 3 crucial elements for effective weight reduction. They also include lots of vitamins and minerals.

4. Become more active
Being active is crucial to losing weight and keeping it off. As well as giving loads of health advantages, exercise may help burn off the extra calories you cannot reduce via diet alone.

Find an exercise you like and can include it in your schedule.

5. Drink lots of water
People may mistake thirst with hunger. You might wind up ingesting additional calories when a glass of water is actually what you need.

Read more about drinking water as part of a healthy diet

6. Eat high-fiber foods

Foods with plenty of fiber may help keep you feeling full, which is excellent for reducing weight. Fiber is exclusively found in meals from plants, such as fruit and veg, oats, wholegrain bread, brown rice and pasta, and beans, peas, and lentils.

## 7. Read food labels

Knowing how to read food labels might help you pick healthier alternatives. Use the calorie information to find out how a specific item fits into your daily calorie allocation on the weight reduction plan.

Find out more about reading food labels

## 8. Use a smaller plate

Using smaller dishes might help you consume lesser servings. By utilizing smaller plates and bowls, you may be able to gradually get acclimated to eating smaller quantities without becoming hungry. It takes around 20 minutes for the stomach to inform the brain it's full, so eat carefully and stop eating before you feel full.

## 9. Do not restrict meals

Do not prohibit any foods from your weight reduction regimen, particularly the ones you enjoy. Banning foods will simply make you desire them more. There's no reason you cannot enjoy the odd pleasure as long as you keep it under your daily calorie restriction.

## 10. Do not stock unhealthy food

To prevent temptation, do not have junk food – such as chocolate, cookies, crisps, and sugary fizzy drinks – at home. Instead, go for nutritious snacks, such as fruit, unsalted rice cakes, oat cakes, unsalted or unsweetened popcorn, and fruit juice.

## 11. Cut down on booze

A regular glass of wine may have as many calories as a piece of chocolate. Over time, drinking too much may easily lead to weight gain.

12. Plan your meals
Try to plan your breakfast, lunch, supper, and snacks for the week, ensuring you keep to your calorie allotment. You may find it useful to develop a weekly shopping list.

Chapter2

Sharpen your cooking routine and talents

Eating healthily is not restricted to just what you are ingesting. It also has a lot to do with the way of cooking. There are so many various cooking techniques, such as baking, grilling, roasting, smoking, boiling, steaming, frying, and braising, giving you lots of alternatives to select from, but not all are favorable to weight reduction and a healthy lifestyle.

Understanding the different ways you may prepare your favorite meals might help you remain on plan and get one step closer to your objectives while still enjoying yourself this summer. Keep reading to discover more about the best cooking ways to lose weight.

Grilling and Broiling
Summer is the best time for grilling, particularly in South Florida, making the backyard barbecue a crucial feature of the season here. Cooking over open flames provides your favorite but basic items with a special taste.

Grilling is a type of cooking that uses dry heat applied to the surface of the meal. It exposes food to direct heat, generally from below the surface. Grilling is a healthy cooking method because it enables fat to melt and drip from the food being cooked. This is why grilled meats are often fewer in calories than the same meat cooked in frying oil. It is crucial not to charge or cause your food to come in touch with direct flame as this may induce the production of possible carcinogens. Additionally, you may limit your hazards by always cooking on a clean barbecue.

Similar to grilling, broiling is another way of cooking that exposes food to direct heat. Broiling employs high heat from a direct flame to rapidly cook food surfaces, which need little to no oil, thereby lowering calories in your meal.

Baking
Baking is another wonderful form of cooking that cuts down on your fat and calorie consumption, which helps you remain on track and maintain a healthy weight and diet. Baking is a dry-heat cooking technique that is common in an oven. Again, similar to grilling and broiling, baking needs little or no extra oil, minimizing the risk of heart disease and other health concerns.

Baking aids persons who desire to keep a healthy lifestyle. Being on a meal plan doesn't have to be dull. Baking captures the distinct tastes of all the components included in the dish, making the finished baked meal tasty.

Steaming
Steaming may be one of the greatest cooking techniques for conserving nutrients. For example, one research revealed that steaming did not produce any substantial loss of vitamin C compared to the other cooking techniques. While the main negative of steaming veggies is that they may come out bland, there are methods to enhance flavor using herbs and salt.

Sauté\sSautéing is a common way of cooking that employs a tiny quantity of oil in a shallow pan over medium to high heat. According to Blue Zones, sautéing maintains more nutrients than boiling and delivers cardiovascular advantages.

Cuts of meat, fish, and vegetables are suitable possibilities for sautéing. Adding your favorite fresh herbs and spices may go a long way and bring a significant amount of flavor to your dish.

Cooking Method to Avoid: Frying

You can discover that frying food is tasty but is it beneficial for you? It genuinely may potentially be the worst and unhealthiest manner of cooking. A meal that is fried gets higher in calories since the food absorbs the fat of the oils it's being cooked in. Fried meals are also often rich in trans fat, a kind of unsaturated fat. Trans fat has been related to an increased risk of various ailments, such as diabetes, heart disease, and obesity.

Chapter3

Why fast weight loss isn't the best

Though the attraction of the "lose 5 pounds in a week" diet myth is great, there are several reasons why quick shedding may work against your best weight loss attempts.

First, when individuals lose weight abruptly, particularly through fad or crash diets, they are often unable to sustain it because the weight they lose is frequently more muscle mass and water and less fat mass compared to persons who lose weight gradually.
Maintaining lean muscle is vital in weight reduction because it plays a major role in metabolism," says certified health coach and author of Sugar Shock and Beyond Sugar Shock Connie Bennett. "Muscle helps you burn more calories. But when you lose weight too rapidly, you lose muscle and your body slows down calorie burning. Fast

weight reduction may also cause an irreversible slowdown of metabolism."

Rapid weight reduction typically leads to the dreaded yo-yo weight cycling that persistent dieters encounter. A study of previous competitors on NBC's weight reduction television program "The Biggest Loser" revealed the more pounds fell fast, the more the participant's metabolism decreased. The research also indicated that the candidates recovered a large portion of their lost weight in the six years after the competition.

Another Australian research of 200 participants in The Lancet reported that although dieters in the study lost the same amount of weight, the group that lost weight slowly lost 10% more body fat and 50% less lean muscle than the quick weight loss group.

Further exacerbating the situation, when individuals lose weight fast, hunger generally rises while metabolism drops, making it extremely tough to keep the pounds off. Research in Obesity indicates our systems drive us to consume 100 calories more each day for every pound lost. Popular fad diets also very frequently result in vitamin deficits. "And quick weight loss—especially when you limit carbs—is generally entirely water," "What's more, if daily calories are low, the body may also utilize muscle mass as fuel, further decreasing metabolism, since muscle mass is metabolically active."

The bottom line: Shedding weight sensibly is the way to proceed. Experts usually say a safe rate is losing around half a pound to 2 pounds a week. With that objective in mind, here are five tried-and-true techniques to reduce pounds and keep them off for good

Chapter4

Best recommendations for safe and maintenance of weight loss

1. Implement Long-Term Lifestyle and Behavior Changes
When attempting to reduce weight, prohibit the phrase "diet," recommends Albertson. Dieting may be unpleasant and make you hungry, so you continuously think about food, which is precisely what you don't want while attempting to lose weight. Instead, she advocates thinking of weight reduction as a component of being healthy and focused on taking care of your body first.

"Weight reduction is difficult and you don't have absolute control over the number on the scale, but you do have control over what you eat, how much you walk, and other things that affect weight, such as stress and sleep," creating SMART—specific, measurable, attainable, relevant, and time-sensitive—goals and praising yourself when you accomplish them.

2. Focus on the First 5% to 10%
Instead of saying, "I need to lose 25 pounds," and overwhelming yourself with what seems like an impossible goal, look toward the health benefits that can come from even modest weight loss.

"Set smaller, achievable targets," suggests Bennett. "Losing merely 5% to 10% of your total body weight (TBW) may considerably improve your health and lessen your risk for diseases, such as type 2 diabetes, stroke, cardiovascular disease, and some forms of cancer."

3. Reduce Your Intake of Ultra-Processed Carbs and Sweets
Research in the Journal of the American Medical Association suggests what you eat is essential for weight loss.
The pounds will come off more rapidly if you increase the quality of the meals you intake.

"One of the best methods to lose weight is to minimize your consumption of sugar and quickly digested carbohydrates," adds Bennett. "In particular, you want to eliminate or substantially reduce your consumption of high-glycemic-load meals, such as sugary snacks, processed carbohydrates, and soft drinks. When you avoid or cut down on French fries, chips, crackers, and the like, you'll speed up your weight loss."
4. Eat More Plants
Research shows a plant-based diet not only promotes weight loss but is also easier to stick to than a low-calorie diet[5]. Plus, it's nutrient dense and has numerous health benefits.

"Produce aids weight reduction because it's high in fiber and water, which are both calorie-free but take up space in your stomach so you feel full," explains Albertson. Brazilian research discovered a clear association between higher fruit and vegetable intake and better weight loss.

Albertson advocates trying to eat five daily portions of produce to start and build up to seven to nine servings a day. "Start your day with a green smoothie, have a salad or chop up veggies with your lunch and eat fruit for snacks and desserts," she recommends. "For the night, have more stir fries, mix vegetables into your pasta dishes and stir them into soups."

5. Pump Up Your Protein
Increasing your protein intake may help lower hunger and assist avoid the loss of muscle mass.

"Eating roughly 25 to 30 grams of protein—two scoops of protein powder or 4 ounces of chicken breast—per meal will enhance appetite control and regulate your body weight," adds Dr. Albertson. "The

easiest way to accomplish that is to make sure you eat one serving of high-quality protein every meal."
women older than 50 need much more protein (1 to 1.5 grams per kilogram of body weight daily) than men and younger women (who need .8 grams of protein per kilogram of body weight daily) (who require .8 grams of protein per kilogram of body weight daily). "Women require extra protein after 50, particularly as they approach menopause since declines in the hormone estrogen result in a loss of skeletal muscle mass, strength, and regeneration ability,

6. Drink More Water

Research showed drinking more water is connected with weight reduction regardless of food and activity. Ample water consumption might assist in promoting satiety and preventing sugar cravings. Water is also important for lipolysis, the body's process of burning fat for energy.

"I advocate following the eight by eight rule—8 ounces of water eight times throughout the day—for a minimum water consumption recommendation," says Florida-based celebrity trainer Jordan Morello who works for the fitness website Sweat Factor. "My customers are frequently shocked once they include this [rule] into their routine [by] how much this simple item can suppress cravings and leave you more full throughout the day."

Another water trick? Try drinking two cups of water before each meal. Studies have shown this simple move can increase weight loss as well.

7. Eat a Well-Rounded Breakfast
Breakfast skippers, listen up. If you're attempting to lose weight, skimping on morning food is not the way to go. Research repeatedly demonstrates missing breakfast is connected with overweight and obesity

Additionally, research in the Proceedings of the Nutrition Society indicated persons who don't have breakfast tend to have worse quality diets overall, and they scrimp on minerals, such as vitamin D, calcium, and iron.

But not just any breakfast will do. "To think more clearly, operate more effectively and be in better moods, you want a well-rounded, blood-sugar-balanced first meal of the day with adequate protein, healthy fats, and what I call quality carbohydrates like fresh berries.

8. Stand Up and Move More
One of the quickest methods to lose weight is to boost your non-exercise activity thermogenesis (NEAT)—the energy spent on everything you do outside of eating, sleeping, or exercising. Little modifications like carrying your goods instead of pushing a cart, parking further away from the entrance to the mall, using the stairs instead

of the elevator, or simply tapping your toe may contribute to hundreds of additional calories burnt.

Or try to stand more than you sit. Studies show that simply replacing sitting with standing leads to a greater daily energy expenditure, which directly translates into more calories burned and ultimately pounds shed.
For example, if you weigh 160 pounds and alternate sitting and standing, you can burn approximately 35 additional calories an hour—an extra 280 calories a day, 1,400 calories a week, and about 70,000 calories a year.

"Set a timer on your phone, Fitbit, or computer to remind you to get up and walk about every hour," adds Albertson. "You'll burn more calories and may lower your blood sugar and risk of heart disease."

9. Hit the Weights
Muscle burns more calories than fat. So how do you build more muscle? Strength training.

Adding resistance training to your weight loss plan is a smart idea not only because of the calories you'll burn while working out but also because of the "afterburn effect."

Known as excess post-exercise oxygen consumption, EPOC reflects how long oxygen uptake remains elevated after exercise to help muscles recover. This rise enhances metabolism both during and after strength exercise sessions.
And the more muscle you put into your physique, the greater your resting metabolic rate (RMR) (RMR). Your RMR determines how many calories your body needs to operate at rest. The greater your RMR, the more you can eat and not gain weight.

"While cardiovascular exercise is often emphasized, strength training is key for dropping pounds and maintaining weight loss, especially after age 50 because muscle mass—which burns calories—declines at a rate of 1% to 2% per year," says Albertson. "Strength training may slow down muscle mass decline."

10. Don't Go Overboard
Cutting calories too drastically or working out 24/7 may backfire when it comes to weight loss. Most people think shedding pounds requires draconian measures to get results but allowing yourself adequate recovery time is more productive.

"Many individuals, when they are angry that they haven't lost weight, will double down on the stressor (i.e. catabolic phase) that they are doing," "For example, they'll run more kilometers, double up on the amount of time they spend at the gym and/or consume less food. However, all of the effects we seek from practicing the aforementioned activities occur during the anabolic recovery phase." During the anabolic phase, the body creates muscle mass and eliminates fat mass while recuperating from the stressor, So, instead of pushing yourself to a breaking point, which ends up leading to overtraining and poor outcomes, invest as much focus into rest and nutrition as you do into exercises. " To produce sustained outcomes, attempt to balance your ratio of stress to recuperation.

11. Check in With an Accountability Partner
Sometimes losing weight might seem lonely, but you don't have to do it all by yourself.

Research demonstrates being responsible works. In one research, two-thirds of individuals who entered a weight reduction program with friends maintained their weight loss for six months after the sessions ended, compared to only a quarter of those who went on their own. Of course, many organizations also advocate having a sponsor or champion on your route to weight reduction.

"One of the greatest ways to regularly eat healthier and reduce weight slowly is to check in every day with an accountability partner," recommends Bennett. "Your accountability buddy doesn't need to be your bestie, favorite co-worker, or lover. Just locate someone with comparable weight reduction objectives. You don't need to chat every day, either. Just text each other to report that you're eating healthy meals and remaining on track. If you're tempted by unhealthy foods, you may count on your spouse, too. That's when you may wish to contact them."

12. Watch Less Television
Couch surfers trying to lose weight should switch off the TV the more television individuals watch, the more weight they acquire.

One research that gathered data from more than 50,000 middle-aged women over six years revealed that for every two hours the participants spent watching television each day, they had a 23% greater chance of obesity and a 14% higher risk of acquiring diabetes.
Excess television viewing is connected with excess pounds largely because it's a sedentary pastime that frequently often leads to thoughtless eating. So, turn it off or maybe change the channel to an exercise program instead.

13. Reconnect With Your Satiety Cues
Speaking of mindless eating, you can rewire your brain for weight reduction by tuning back into your body's natural "I'm hungry" and "I'm full" signals.


"Dieting paired with eating on the fly or while multitasking—driving, watching TV, playing with your phone—can completely separate you from your normal signals of hunger and satiety," adds Albertson. "Plus, as youngsters, we are also taught to clear our plates rather than eat until satisfied." Add the fact that portion sizes have expanded significantly—as much as 60% for items like snack foods— and the effect is continuous overeating.

"Instead, aim to eat when you're hungry and end when you are content rather than stuffed," adds Albertson. "Instead of monitoring your food, consider measuring how hungry you feel before, during, and after meals to get back in touch with these signals."

14. Get More Sleep

Getting a good night's sleep is one of the finest things you can do to maintain a healthy weight and general health. Studies demonstrate that inadequate sleep is related to weight gain and other health concerns. When researchers studied 16

years' worth of data on 68,183 middle-aged
American women, they discovered those
who slept little more than five hours each
night were 15% more likely to develop
obesity compared to those who slept seven
hours a night.
Insufficient sleep may also impact the
production of appetite-regulating hormones
ghrelin and leptin, which may cause
individuals to feel hungry during the day.
Additionally, poor sleep boosts cortisol and
might result in a harder-to-lose body and
belly fat.

"Most of us can't control what time we have
to get up, but we can control when we go to
bed, so counting back seven to nine hours
from the time you have to wake up is a great
tip, "I also encourage the 3-2-1 rule, which
means stop working three hours before bed,
stop eating two hours before bed and stop
digital stimuli one hour before bed to
improve your deep sleep and REM."

## 15. Find Non-Edible Substitutes for Self-Soothing

There's a reason it's called "comfort food." However, emotional eating may easily undermine any weight reduction attempts.

"When you feel stressed, which raises cortisol levels, rather than reaching for food to feel better—since eating triggers the release of the feel-good neurotransmitter dopamine—raise levels of oxytocin, the love hormone, either by soothing touch, playing with a pet or getting a hug.

Animal studies have found oxytocin reduces calories consumed and has positive effects on metabolism[15]. A small human study also found that giving men oxytocin over eight weeks promoted weight loss. While more research is needed to understand exactly how increasing oxytocin can impact weight and appetite, if you're experiencing difficult emotions, a self-compassion break will allow you to give yourself the care you need so you will be less likely to eat," says Albertson. "Remember the acronym 'HALT,' which stands for hungry, angry/anxious, lonely, and tired. If you are physiologically hungry, eat. If you are feeling tough emotions, ask, 'What do I need?' and offer yourself what you genuinely need. If you're not hungry, it isn't food."

www.ingramcontent.com/pod-product-compliance
Lightning Source LLC
Chambersburg PA
CBHW072331270726
48658CB00016B/2325